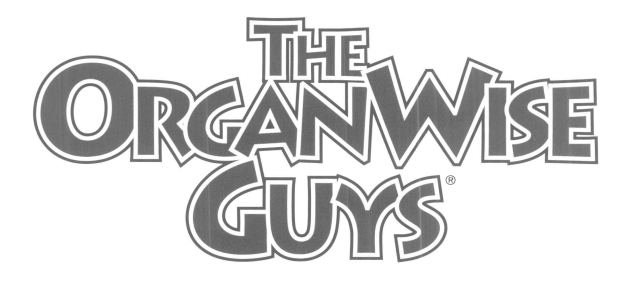

## Basic Training for Better Health

written by
Michelle Lombardo, D.C.

illustrated by
M.R. Herron

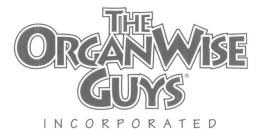

INCORPORATED

Copyright © 1999, 2006 by The OrganWise Guys Incorporated, 3838 Song River Circle, Duluth, GA 30097 Phone (800) 786-1730
www.organwiseguys.com

# HI THERE!

I'm HARDY HEART. I am the leader of THE ORGANWISE GUYS. Some of you may know about our club and some may even be members! We teach kids all about being smart from the inside out. Well, whether or not you know about our club really shouldn't matter at this point because something even more exciting has happened to us! Washington, D.C. has found out about The OrganWise Guys and has started a nationwide program with me as the leader!

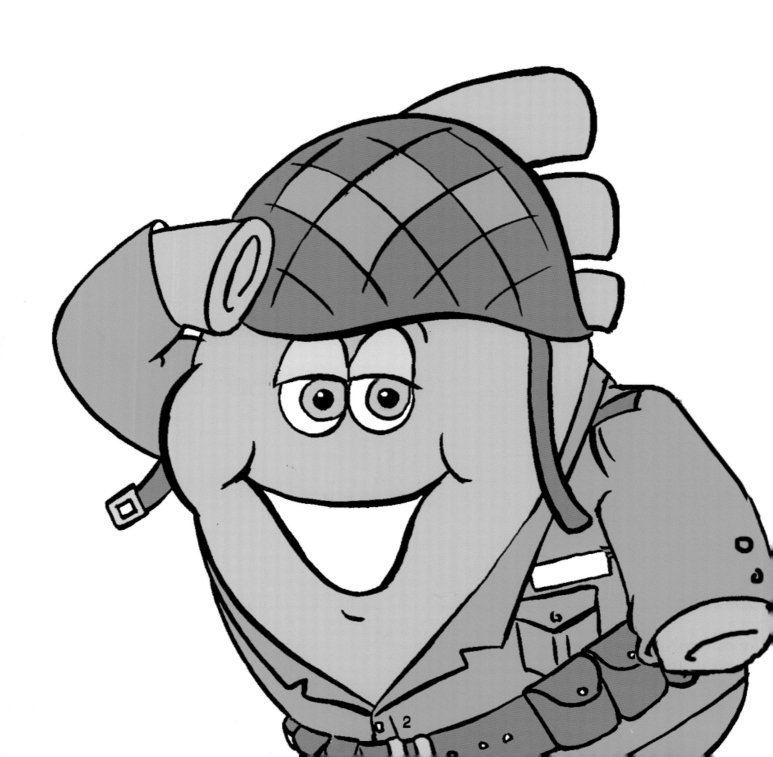

# I WANT YOU. . .WELL!

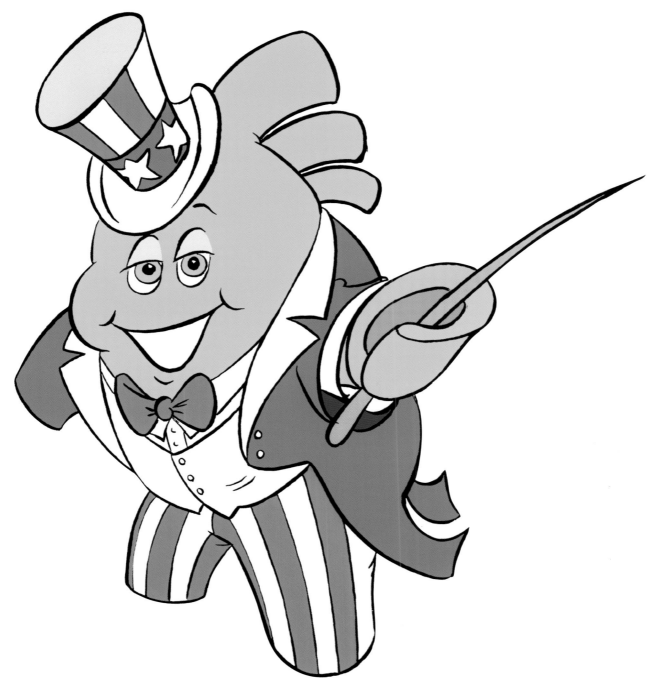

My mission is to teach new recruits about making changes for a healthier tomorrow. Here I am in my new, official threads. I travel around the country looking for kids of all ages who are interested in becoming healthier. Remember, I want you . . .well! There are some really easy things that each person can do everyday to fight off sickness and disease. We are just getting ready to form the first platoon of THE ORGANWISE GUYS. I'd like to introduce you to some of the new recruits.

# ATTENTION!

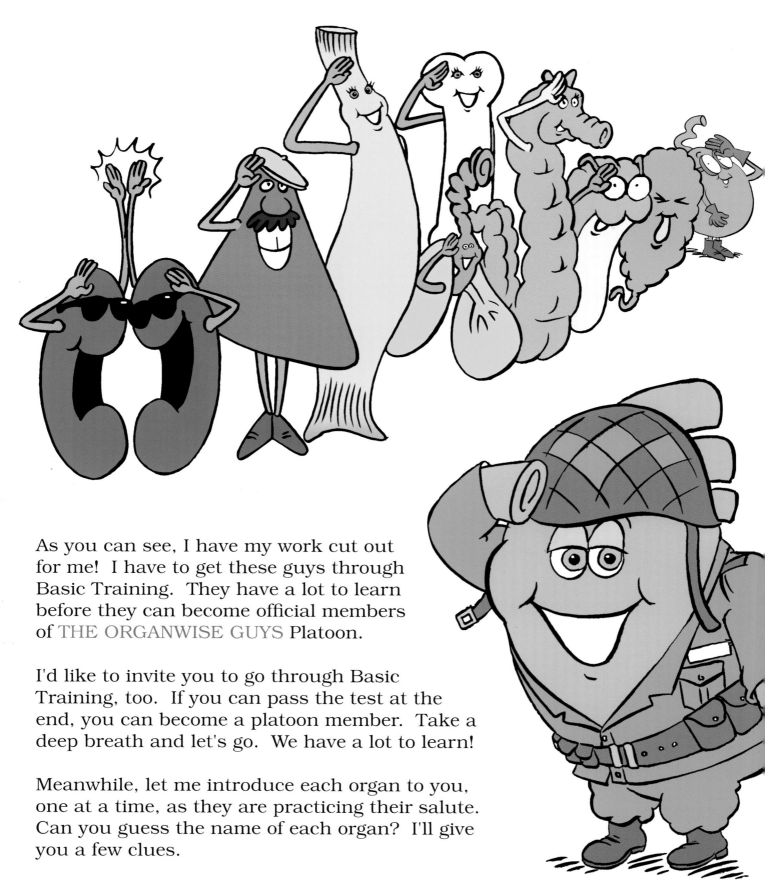

As you can see, I have my work cut out for me! I have to get these guys through Basic Training. They have a lot to learn before they can become official members of THE ORGANWISE GUYS Platoon.

I'd like to invite you to go through Basic Training, too. If you can pass the test at the end, you can become a platoon member. Take a deep breath and let's go. We have a lot to learn!

Meanwhile, let me introduce each organ to you, one at a time, as they are practicing their salute. Can you guess the name of each organ? I'll give you a few clues.

4

# THESE ORGANS BEGIN WITH THE LETTER, "K."

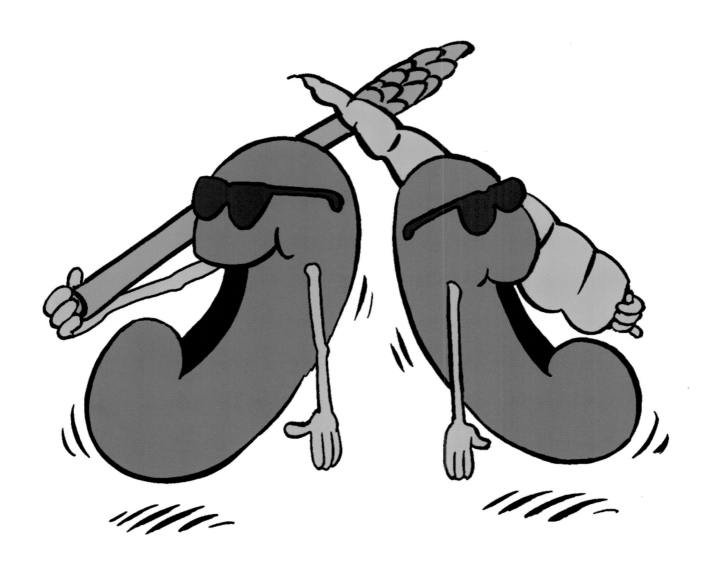

They are the part of the body that is like a water treatment plant. There are two of them and they sit side by side inside your middle back area.

Did you guess, "the kidneys?" These guys are THE KIDNEY BROTHERS. They are twins, Sid and Kid. They like to have a good time! I hope they realize that boot camp can be fun, but it is a lot of hard work, too.

# THIS ORGAN BEGINS WITH THE LETTER, "L."

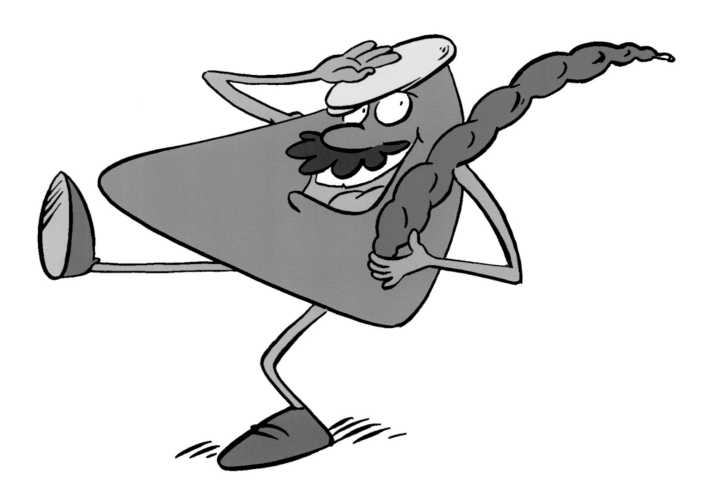

This organ works hard using the food we eat to build a healthier body. It is also the organ that works to get rid of any poisons in the body.

That's right! It's the liver. His name is LUIGI LIVER. He goofs off once in a while, but is usually a serious fellow. I guess it's because he knows what an important job he has keeping the body healthy.

# GUESS WHICH PARTS OF THE BODY THESE ARE?

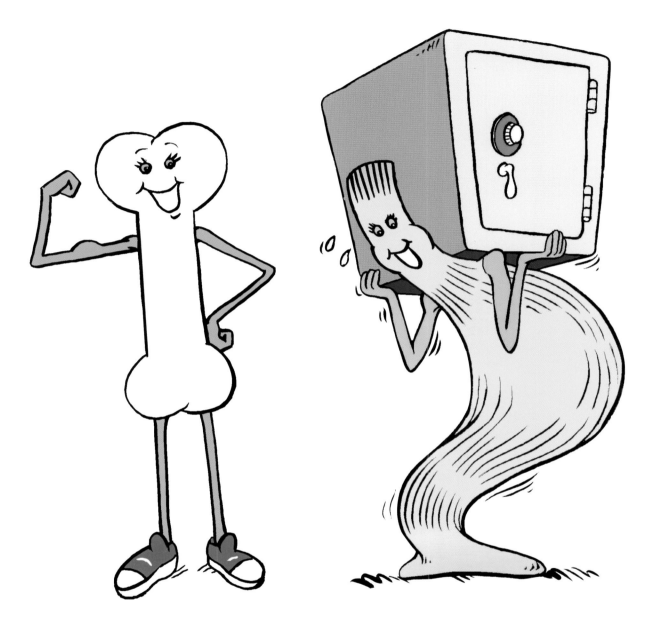

Both of these parts need you to exercise to keep them strong. They are not really organs, but you have a bunch of them in your body. They work together when it comes time to do heavy lifting.

They are CALCI M. BONE and MADAME MUSCLE. They really want to be in the platoon, but at first did not realize how important physical activity was for platoon members. They didn't think sweating was something girls should do - that is until they both learned about the importance of staying fit!

# THIS ORGAN BEGINS WITH THE LETTER, "L."

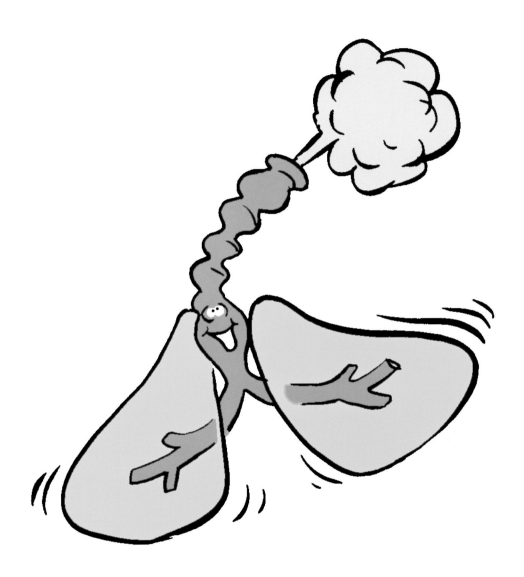

This part of the body needs a lot of healthy, fresh air. The thing that really hurts this organ is the foolish habit of smoking cigarettes.

I knew you would get this right! It's the lungs. Her name is WINDY. She got her name because of her "windpipe." When she is healthy she flies around like a little butterfly. She soars like the wind! It is really important to keep the lungs healthy because this is how you get oxygen to every part of the body.

# THIS PART BEGINS WITH THE LETTER, "I."

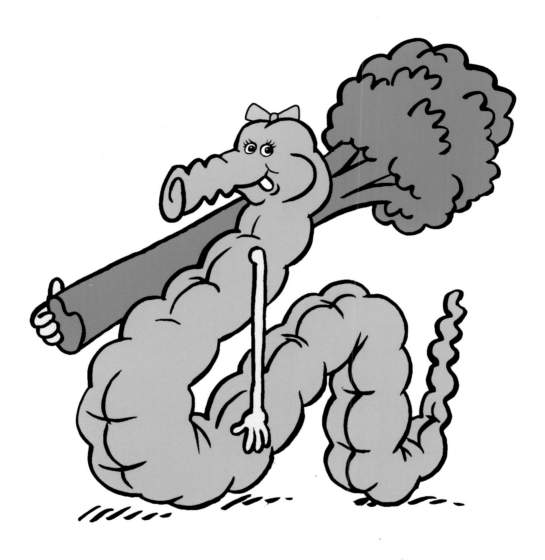

This organ is like a long, squiggly worm. It is the last part of your digestive system. It's the intestine.

The intestine is very important because it's where a lot of nutrients are absorbed for the body to use. Her name is PERI STOLIC. People may laugh at her because of her job. But once they learn how important and nice she is, they realize how mean it is to make fun of someone. All of the other recruits really like Peri and if anyone says anything bad about her, they better watch out!

# THIS ONE IS A NO-BRAINER. . .

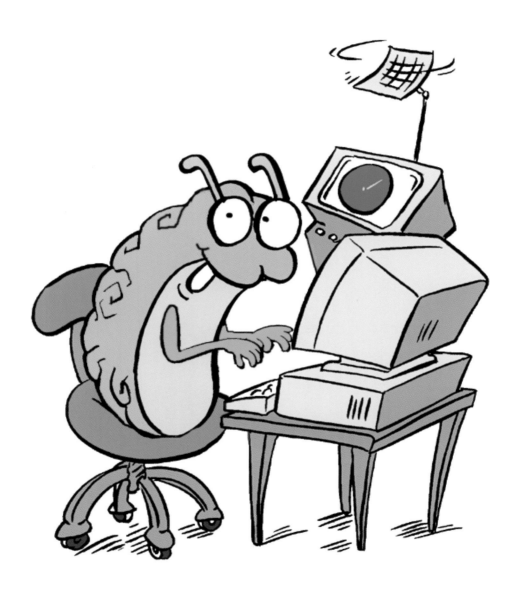

This organ is kind of like a computer. It controls the rest of the body through nerves. That's right! It's the brain. His name is SIR REBRUM. His name sounds like one of the brain parts, the cerebrum. He is a really smart guy.

# THIS ORGAN BEGINS WITH THE LETTER, "P."

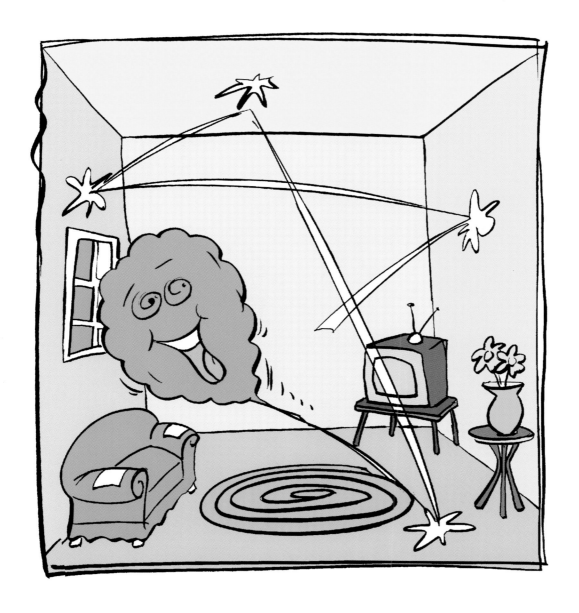

This part of the body helps keep the blood sugar levels under control. It makes insulin, which is very important. He is not a really popular organ, but he is very important in keeping us alive. I'll be shocked if you guess it!

This is the pancreas. His name is PETER PANCREAS. Like all of us, he sometimes gets a little wild and crazy. Once in a while the others have to tell him to try and calm down before he bounces off the wall. I'll bet with all of his energy he will be great during the exercise portion of Basic Training!

# THIS PART OF YOUR BODY BEGINS WITH THE LETTER, "S."

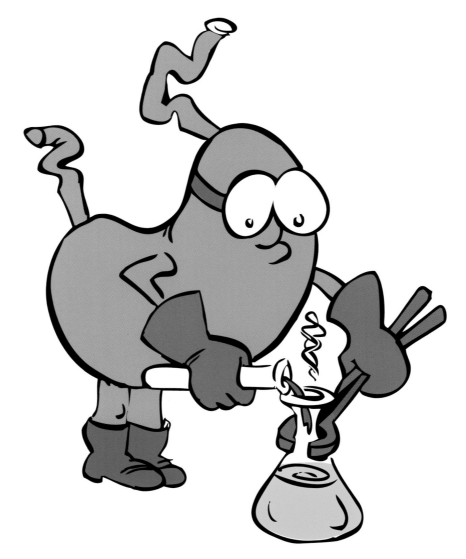

This final organ makes juices to help digest food. One of the main juices is "pepsin." This organ also has muscles in it to help mash the food, and it is where the food goes when you first eat it.

You've got it! It's the stomach. His name is PEPTO because of the pepsin. Now Pepto is the nervous type. THE ORGANWISE GUYS are trying to teach Pepto not to worry so much and enjoy life a little more. I'll bet he is a little uptight about getting into the platoon. I'm sure if he will do his best, he'll be just fine.

# PLATOON RULES:

1. REGULAR EXERCISE
2. EAT A LOW-FAT DIET
3. EAT A HIGH-FIBER DIET
4. DRINK PLENTY OF WATER

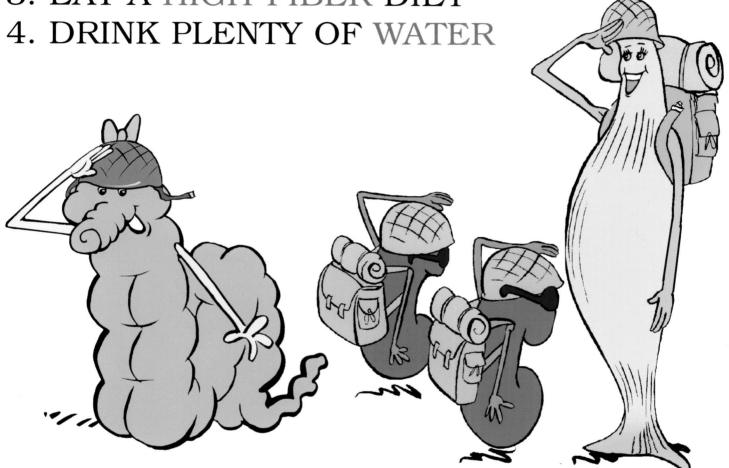

The first thing we need to go over are the platoon rules. Make sure you study these because all new recruits need to know them. Let's say the words in RED aloud as if we are in boot camp. Remember to say "Sir" at the end of each one.

READY NEW RECRUITS:　EXERCISE, SIR
　　　　　　　　　　　　LOW-FAT, SIR
　　　　　　　　　　　　HIGH-FIBER, SIR
　　　　　　　　　　　　WATER, SIR

Hey, that sounded pretty good!

# THE ENEMY OF YOUR BODY IS. . .

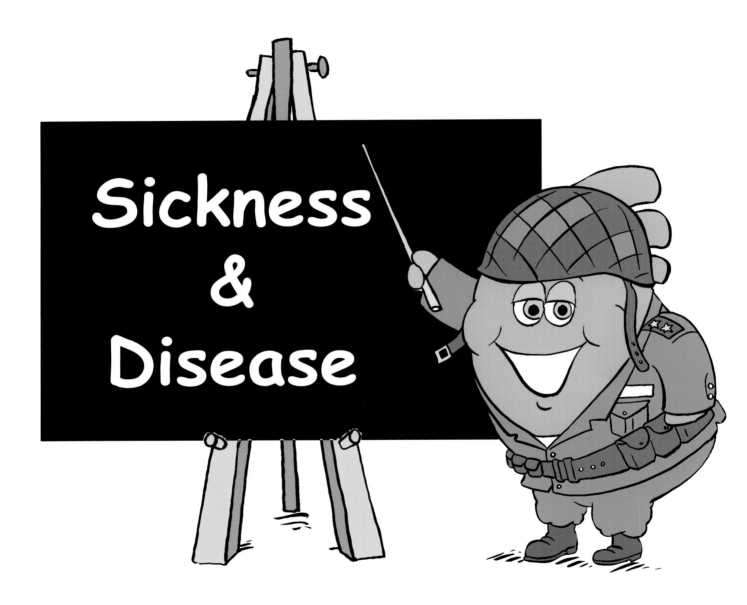

Our next step is to *know the enemy*. We are in a battle to keep your body healthy. A lot of kids think that when a germ gets in the body, you automatically get sick. It doesn't have to always be that way. We are going to be looking at ways that you can help your body attack sickness instead of it attacking you! Let's take a closer look at one of the culprits that can make you sick.

# A CLOSER LOOK. . .

This is the dreaded cold bug or germ. As you can see, I have to use a microscope because these things are so small. Have your parents ever told you to stay away from someone who has a cold so you won't catch it? These are the little guys they are talking about. The good news is, the body has a defense system to attack these invaders. Let's take a closer look at what I am talking about.

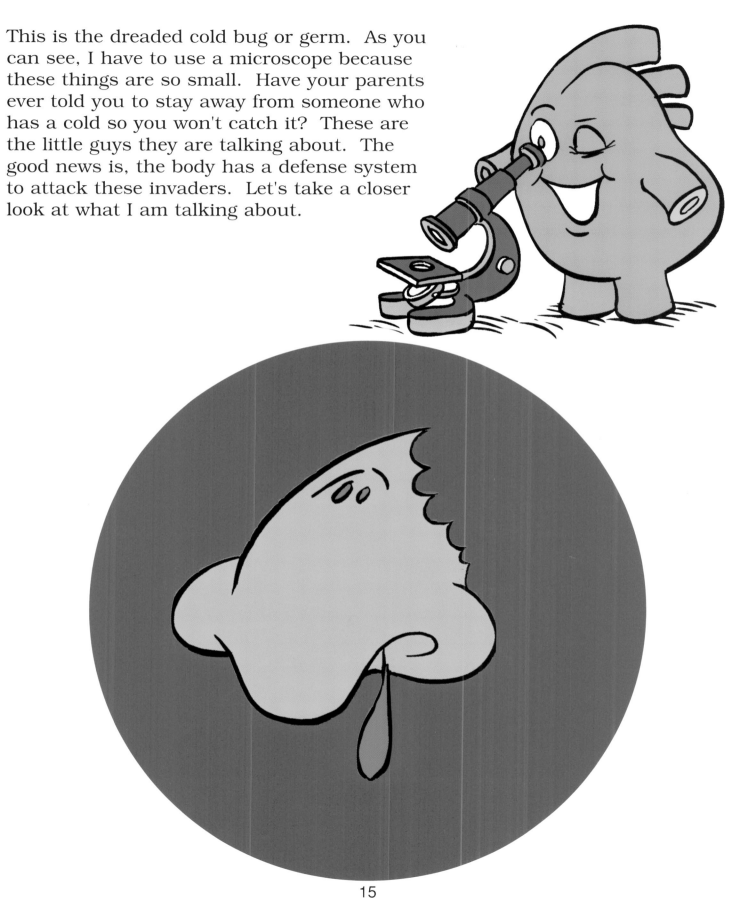

# THE COMMON COLD. . .

The cold bug has found your body and it is ready to give you a cold. But don't panic! Have you ever heard of your immune system? Do you see these "T" soldiers? These are called T-CELLS. They are like soldiers that find these bad guys and flag them. Now the germs are ready for the next step in their destruction. . .

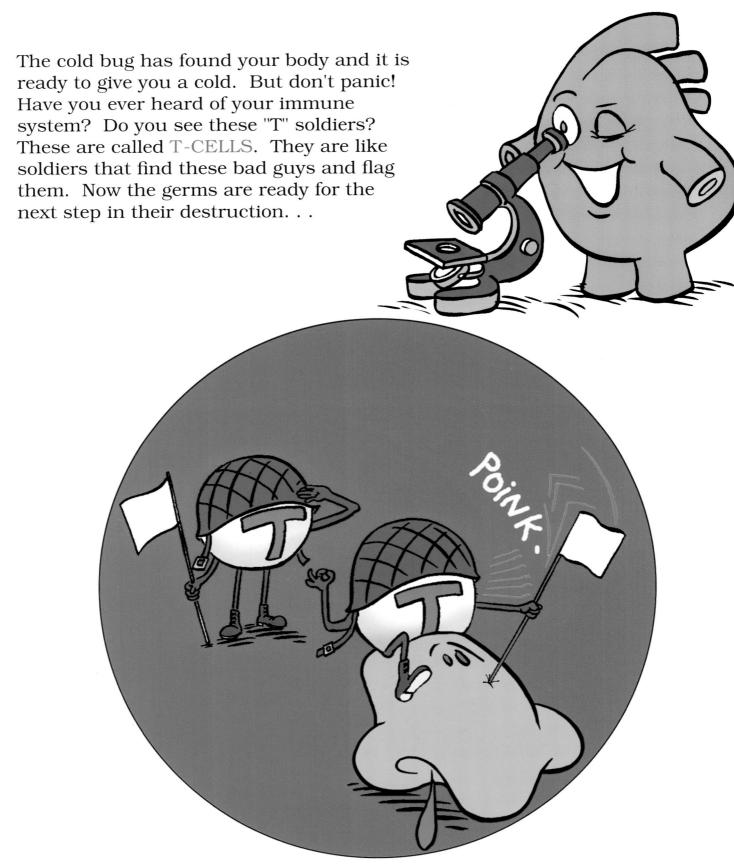

# THE GOOD GUYS. . .

. . . It's the attack of the WHITE BLOOD CELLS! The white blood cells are like eating machines. They see the cold bug with the flag and guess what they do? That's right, they eat 'em! I think it is really amazing how the body works. How can you help your immune system?

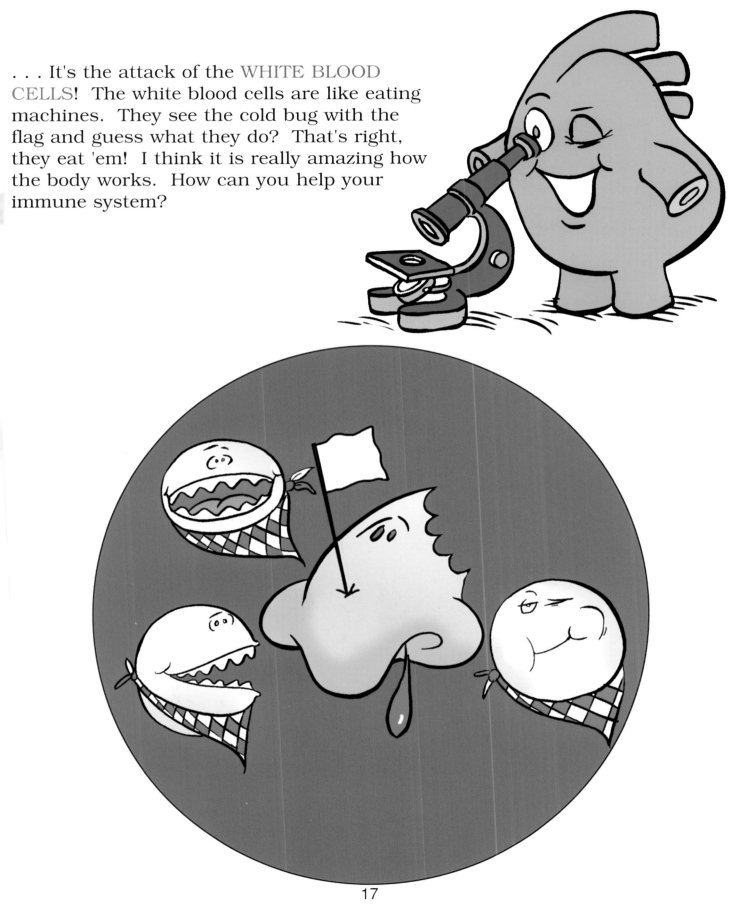

# RULE #1. . .EXERCISE!

Do you remember rule number one?  It is regular EXERCISE.  Let's see why it is so important.

When you do regular exercise, it builds up your immune system.  Think of it as exercising your T-CELLS AND WHITE BLOOD CELLS.  They run around inside of you looking for the germs.  This is why people who exercise regularly don't get sick as much.

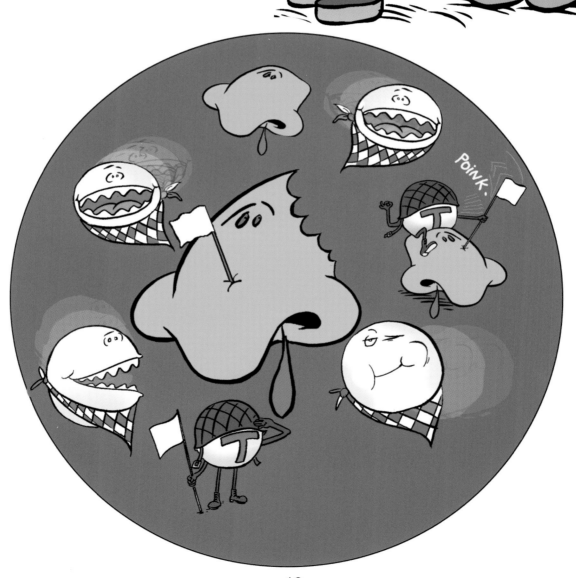

# RULE #2. . . .EAT LOW-FAT!

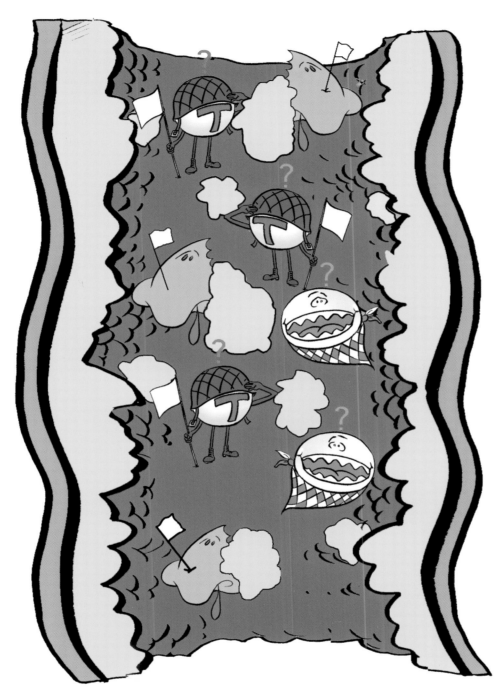

The next plan of attack, new recruits, is to make LOW-FAT choices. Let's take a look inside the artery of someone who eats lots of fried food, butter, and other high-fat foods every single day. Do you see all the yellow stuff in the blood? That is fat! When you have a lot of fat in your blood, the blood is really thick. The germs like it this way because they can hide in the fat. Now the T-CELLS and the WHITE BLOOD CELLS can't find the germs and destroy them. The germs can sneak around and make the body sick.

# IT'S YOUR CHOICE. . .

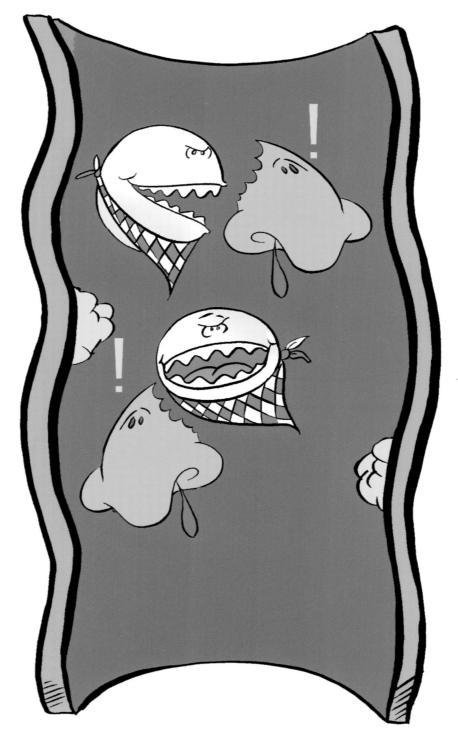

Now let's take a look inside the artery of someone who eats high-fat foods once in a while (we all do that), but who also makes low-fat choices. Do you see much fat in their artery? Guess what's going to happen to the germs?

That's right! The white blood cells are going to eat them. Who thinks they need to start making low-fat choices?

# FREE RADICALS. . .

Now I need to tell you about another one of the culprits that likes to damage the human body. This guy is called a FREE RADICAL. He looks pretty radical, huh? Do you see the thing swirling around his head? It is an electron. Now I am teaching college stuff here, so listen up! This free radical doesn't like having just one electron. He wants to steal another one from a healthy cell in your body. But don't worry - there is a way to get rid of this thief!

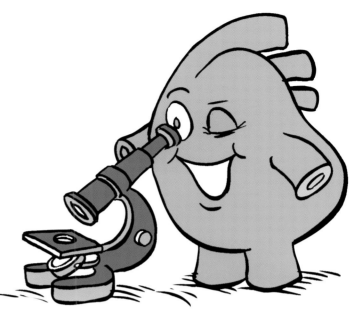

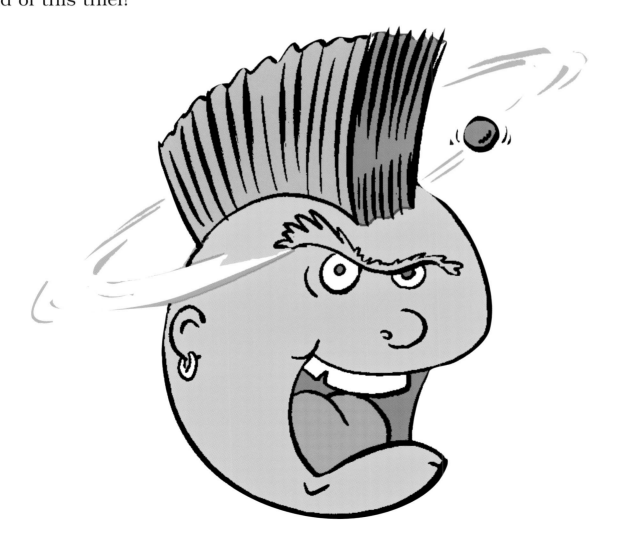

# RULE #3. . .HIGH-FIBER!

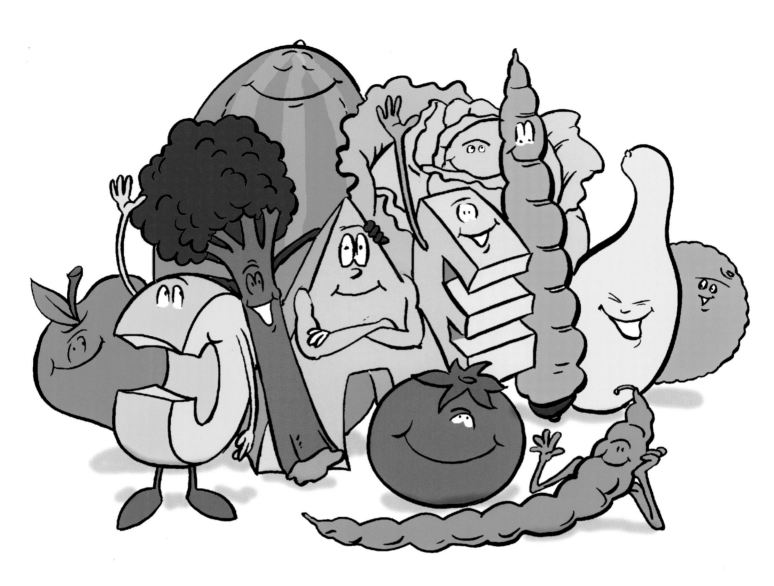

This brings us to the third plan of attack, new recruits. We need to eat high-fiber foods like fruits and vegetables! These foods help the intestines work better. Also, when kids (and their parents) eat fruits and veggies they are getting important vitamins called ANTI-OXIDANTS. I know it is a big word so let me make it easier for you. Can you spot the antioxidant vitamins in these fruits and vegetables?

That's right. VITAMINS A, C, & E. An easy way to remember this is by saying the word ACE. Let me show you what these ACE vitamins do to the free radicals after kids eat their fruits and vegetables.

# LOCK 'EM UP. . .

Once these vitamins get into the blood, they hook up with the free radicals so they can't steal electrons from your healthy cells.  I like to think of these vitamins as policemen locking up the thieves.  So, new recruits, who thinks they need to be eating more fruits and vegetables?  I do, too!

# RULE #4. . .
# DRINK WATER!

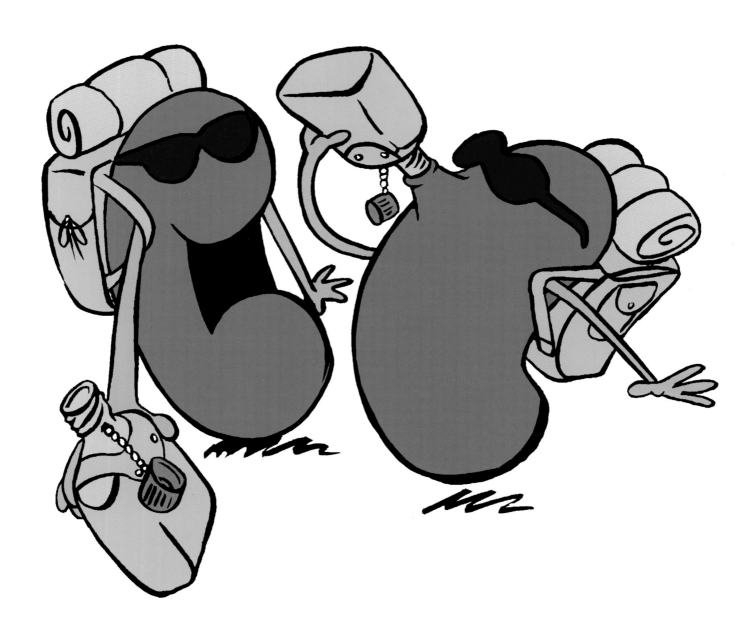

The final plan of attack is to drink lots of WATER. The kidney's main job is to filter the blood and help keep it clean. Just like a water treatment plant, it needs water to work. Please, please, please give your kidneys plenty of fluids, especially water! And remember, the more you exercise, the more you sweat and the more you need to drink fluids.

# READ THE LABELS. . .

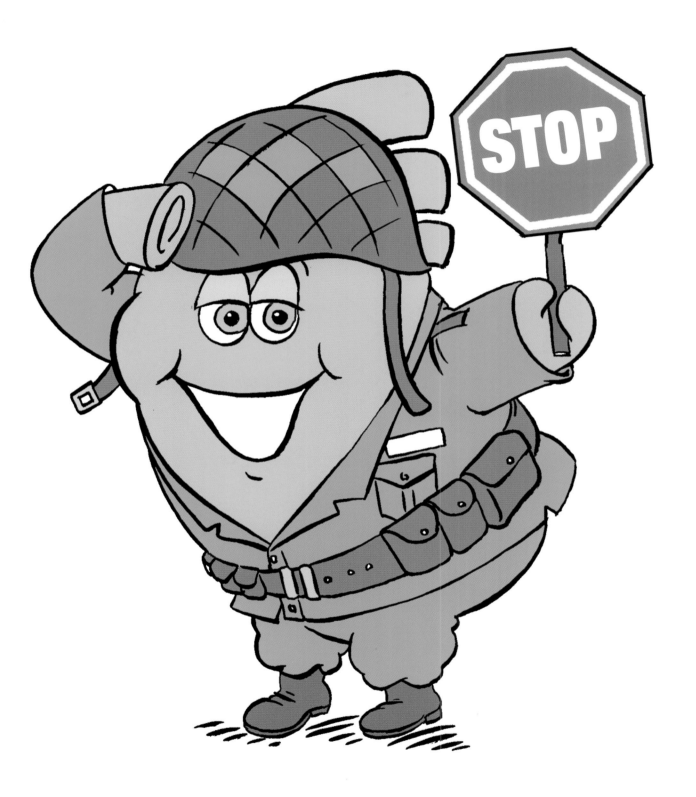

Your mission, new recruits, is to start with one easy step towards better health.  You need to STOP AND READ THE LABELS!  How do you read labels?  It's easy. . .

# FOCUS IN. . .

**Nutrition Facts**

Serving Size 8 Wafers (32g)
Servings Per Container About 8

**Amount Per Serving**

**Calories** 130    Calories from Fat 25

| | % Daily Value* |
|---|---|
| **Total Fat** 3g | **5**% |
| Saturated Fat 0.5g | **3**% |
| **Cholesterol** 0mg | **0**% |
| **Sodium** 180mg | **7**% |
| **Total Carbohydrate** 24g | **8**% |
| Dietary Fiber 4g | **17**% |
| Sugars 0g | |
| **Protein** 3g | |

Vitamin A 0% • Vitamin C 0% • Calcium 0%

Iron 10% • Phosphorus 15%

\* Percent Daily Values are based on a 2,000 calorie diet. Your daily values may be higher or lower depending on your calorie needs:

| | | Calories: | 2,000 | 2,500 |
|---|---|---|---|---|
| Total Fat | Less than | | 65g | 80g |
| Sat Fat | Less than | | 20g | 25g |
| Cholesterol | Less than | | 300mg | 300mg |
| Sodium | Less than | | 2400mg | 2400mg |
| Total Carbohydrate | | | 300g | 375g |
| Dietary Fiber | | | 25g | 30g |

I know labels can be confusing. There are numbers all over the place! Just focus in on one item at a time. Start by looking at grams of fat. How many TOTAL FAT grams are there in one serving of these crackers?

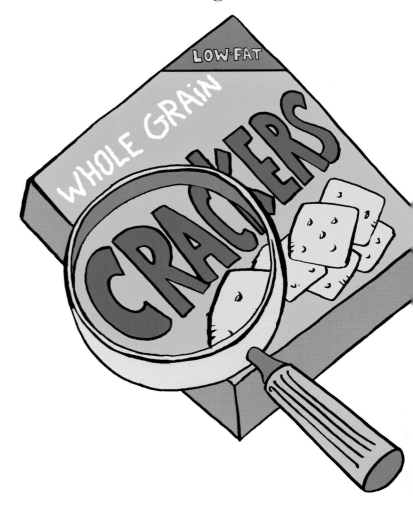

Did you find it? Yes, there are 3 grams of fat. The good news is that once you know how to read one label you can read them all. All the food labels are the same. So start checking the foods you eat for total grams of fat. Make low-fat choices when you can. It's okay to treat yourself to higher fat foods once in awhile, just remember to get plenty of exercise when you do.

Can you find how many total grams of DIETARY FIBER are in one serving of this item? That's right, 4 grams! This seems to fit right in with what THE ORGANWISE GUYS need: a low-fat, high-fiber snack!

# THE CADENCE MARCH. . .

Now, on to my favorite part of boot camp, the cadence march!  The platoon starts each day with exercise.  You know, as a heart, I love that!  We have a song we march to as we go.  The beat follows the, "Left, left, left, right, left" march.  I am sure you have all heard that.  You are not going to believe who leads the recruits . . . that's right, MADAME MUSCLE!  She sings the line first and then the group follows along as they march.

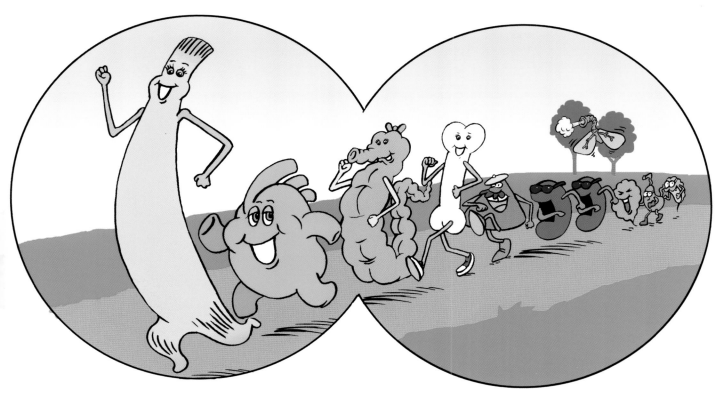

I will try to eat low-fat,
Eating low-fat is where it's at.

High-fiber is what I'll choose,
With fruits and veggies I can't lose.

I'll drink water everyday,
and I'll wash disease away.

Exercise to keep me strong,
With these rules I can't go wrong.

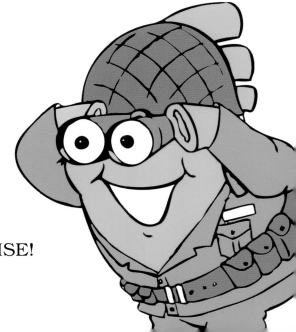

ROLL CALL:
LOW-FAT, HIGH-FIBER, LOTS OF WATER, EXERCISE!

# GREAT JOB. . .

. . . and remember what else is going on inside of you. The T-CELLS and your WHITE BLOOD CELLS are running around fighting germs. Isn't that good news?

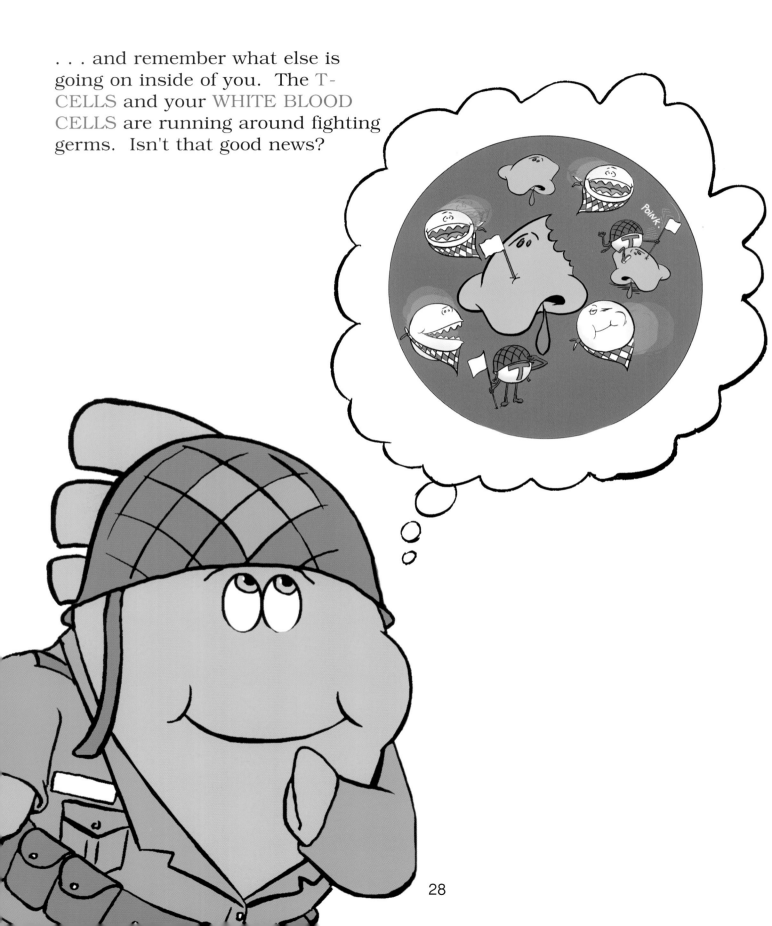

28

# THE TEST. . .

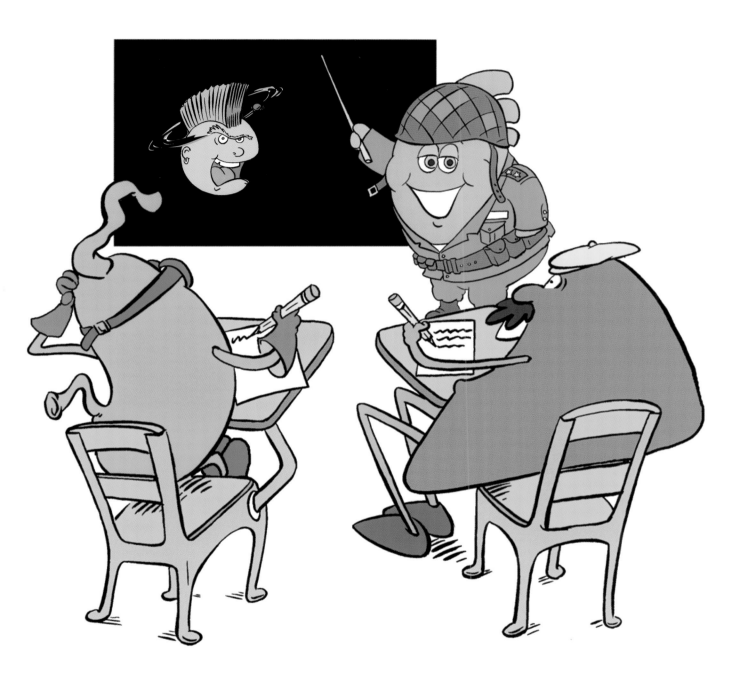

I must say, this platoon has shaped up to be one of the best around! Are you ready for the test? I'm going to be asking you four questions. You need to make sure you say, "Sir" after each answer.

Are you ready? I hope you answered, "YES, SIR!"

# 4 BIG QUESTIONS. . .

NUMBER 1: You need to make sure that your T-CELLS and your white blood cells are running around inside of you fighting the germs. You need to get plenty of what. . .

_____, SIR!

NUMBER 2: You need to make sure there is not a lot of this yellow stuff floating around in your blood where the germs can hide. You need to eat low-something. New recruits, what do you want to eat?

LOW - _____, SIR!

NUMBER 3: You need to make sure you are eating plenty of fruits and veg-etables. Both have lots of vitamins and are high-something. New recruits, you have to eat what?

HIGH - _____, SIR!

NUMBER 4: You need to make sure your kidneys can do their job. You need to drink plenty of fluids. New recruits, what drink do the kidneys like best?

_____, SIR!

COME ON RECRUITS. . .
YOU CAN DO IT!

30

# YOU PASSED!

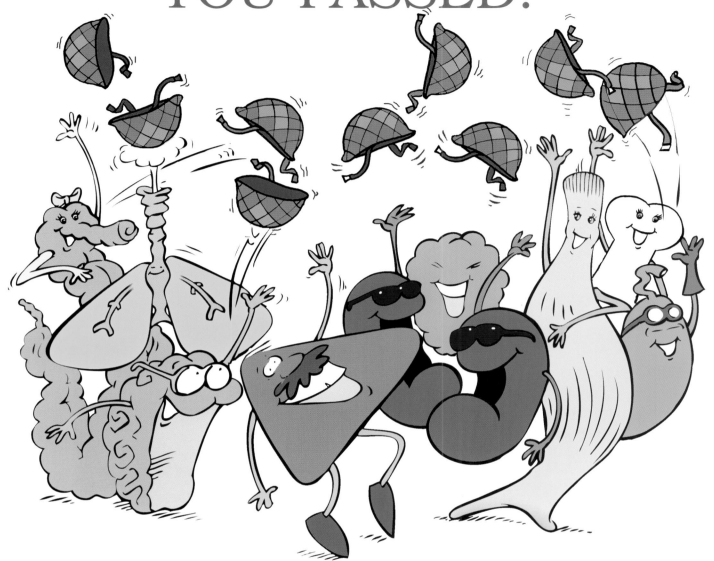

NOW FOR THE FINAL STEP.
RAISE YOUR RIGHT HAND AND REPEAT THE OFFICIAL OATH:

I do solemnly swear.
To try to be healthy.
To eat low-fat.
To eat high-fiber.
To drink more water.
And to get plenty of exercise.
I am proud to be
an official member of
The OrganWise Guys platoon!

# CONGRATULATIONS!

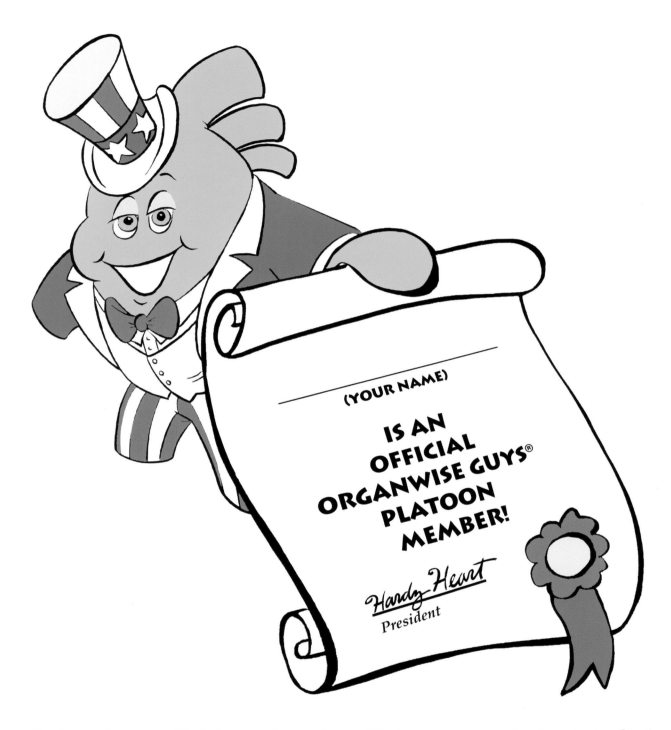

**(YOUR NAME)**

**IS AN OFFICIAL ORGANWISE GUYS® PLATOON MEMBER!**

*Hardy Heart*
President

Now that you're an official member of our Platoon, your mission is to find more recruits! Tell your parents, friends and everyone you know about making low-fat choices, eating high-fiber foods, drinking lots of water and exercising every day.

**REMEMBER, IT'S EVERYBODY'S DUTY TO TAKE CHARGE OF THEIR OWN HEALTH!**